NATURAL ANTI-AGING WISDOM

SECRETS TO LOOK YOUNGER, LIVE LONGER, AND FEEL HEALTHY, WITHOUT A DOCTOR'S PRESCRIPTION

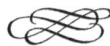

JOHN GIANETTI

CONTENTS

Natural Anti-Aging Wisdom	v
Introduction	vii
1. Three Things You Can Immediately Implement To Look & Feel Younger	1
2. Fitness Tips To Prevent Aging	9
3. The Secret To Keeping Your Mind Young & Healthy	14
Afterword	19

NATURAL ANTI-AGING WISDOM

Secrets to Look Younger, Live Longer, and Feel Healthy, Without a Doctor's Prescription

John Gianetti

INTRODUCTION

This book was designed for people who want to learn about natural ways to stay young, healthy looking, and feel more vibrant. Often times people resort to unnatural ways to in attempts to look younger and end up spending thousands of dollars when it's completely unnecessary!

While reading this you will learn plenty of strategies and tips that are new as well as ones that have been used for many years to keep people looking young and beautiful.

Aging With Beauty

> "Aging is not lost youth but a new stage of opportunity and strength."
>
> -**Betty Friedan**

Each human being has his own fears- fear of being alone, fear of failures, and fear of dying. Each fear represents a person's weakness and your weaknesses remind you that you

INTRODUCTION

are a human being. Being human has a lot of consequences, and one of them is aging. One of the most feared things in this world is the fact that all humans are bound to age and die. This is something that many people want to delay and a process that most people equate with disease and dying. Aging is a normal phenomenon that no human being can ever avoid. But though it is a process that is already expected to happen from the time of birth, many people are still doing everything they can to avoid it. They apply different creams onto their skin, take various medicines, and undergo certain procedures just to prevent aging from happening.

The truth about aging is that it is unavoidable. From the time of conception, aging has already been happening. After fertilization, you develop into a zygote, into an embryo, and then into a fetus. Your cells mature and your organs develop. The reason why many people are afraid of it is because of how they define aging. Some people would think of aging as a normal process that involves maturation and development, while some would think of it as the period of increased risk to certain diseases.

Aging has both positive and negative repercussions. However, more often than not, it is the negative effect of aging that people are most aware and concerned of. Aging is attributed to many factors, such as the genetic and bio physiological factors that govern the processes occurring inside the human body, and the environmental factors that may accelerate the aging process.

One of the most well known theories of aging is the theory on telomeres. Each human being is unique due to his DNA make-up. Science has proven that no two DNA sequences are alike, just like how your fingerprints are different from

INTRODUCTION

other people. Each DNA is made up of two strands of nucleic acids intertwined with each other. At the end of each strand are telomeres that are said to shorten in length every time cell division occurs.

Cell division is the process by which cells produce daughter cells. This is most evident during periods of cell renewal and restoration. For example, you lost a part of your liver due to trauma or disease; your liver cells are stimulated to divide more rapidly, to regenerate and restore what was lost. However, there is greater risk of telomere shortening with higher frequency of cell division.

Telomeres are said to be the part of the human DNA responsible for aging. The length of telomeres is predetermined at birth and telomeres are not capable of elongation, unless an enzyme called telomerase is activated. This telomerase enzyme adds new portions to the telomere and allows the telomere to elongate even with cell division. All individuals have this enzyme, but this is kept in an inactivated state. Telomerase enzyme is said to be activated in cancers, making cell division limitless. Once telomeres are shortened to a certain length, cell division stops and cellular aging occurs.

The generation of free radicals is also a major concern in aging. Experts say that cellular metabolism produces substances that are toxic to the body. These substances are known as free radicals that are said to be damaging to the cells. Free radicals are unpaired electrons that form unstable compounds within the body. They are produced by oxidation- reduction processes that are involved in the generation of energy, inflammation and even infection.

Under normal circumstances, the body fights off these free

radicals with the help of glutathione produced by the liver. Endogenous glutathione serves as a potent antioxidant that neutralizes free radicals and thus, counteracts their damaging effects. However, in times of stress, and exposure to infectious agents and various chemicals, the amount of glutathione being produced by the liver may no longer be enough to neutralize the great amount of free radicals generated.

Stress can stimulate the release of certain hormones, such as adrenaline and nor-adrenaline that increase the rate of metabolic processes in the body. Though the acute release of these hormones is deemed helpful to fight off stress, they might induce harm in the long run causing more production of free radicals. Exposure to infection and chemicals can also cause production of free radicals by stimulating the inflammatory process and increasing the metabolic rate of the body.

Aging affects several aspects in a person's life, such as the physical, mental and social dimensions. Physical changes are the most noticeable and are thus, the major concerns of most people. Older people may start to experience weakness, which is usually manifested as a decrease in the amount of work that they can do. They may no longer be able to carry 10 kilos of rice like they used to. They also start to notice that they can no longer walk for 500 meters like they used to do before. Older people also start to experience blurring of vision, impairment of hearing, and joint pains. More obvious signs of aging include wrinkling of skin, greying of the hair, and exaggeration of the curvature of the thoracic spine called kyphosis.

Mental changes, on the other hand, refer to the decline in the cognitive function of older people. They may experience memory impairment, which may start as difficulty in remembering information recently learned. As aging goes on, more severe mental impairments occur.

Social changes may manifest as a decrease in the number and quality of interpersonal relationships of the persons affected. These social changes are sometimes attributed to the despair of older people when they reach a certain age. They may start isolating themselves from others and may even have some mood swings.

Despite the inevitability of aging, there are ways on how you can delay the aging process. Since aging occurs as a consequence of environmental factors, certain foods, exercises and a positive attitude can all help prevent its acceleration.

THREE THINGS YOU CAN IMMEDIATELY IMPLEMENT TO LOOK & FEEL YOUNGER

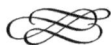

In this day and age, everyone seems to be desperate about finding ways to look younger. People apply various cosmetics just to prevent wrinkles and dark spots from appearing. Although there are many creams, moisturizers and other cosmetics that can effectively reduce these signs of aging, you can opt to go natural and be more cautious of what you eat instead.

1. Drink a lot of water.

60% of the body is made up of water and any imbalance in this level can produce diseases. Hypertension, diabetes mellitus and renal failures all account to an alteration in the fluid levels of the body. Drinking a lot of water does not only prevent the diseases that are most common among the older population, but it also prevents wear and tear of cells.

Water serves many functions in the body. It serves as a transport medium for many nutrients and it also helps in the excretion of by-products of cellular metabolism that are harmful to the body. Water is also needed by the cells in order for them to perform their functions. One of the consequences of lack of water intake is dehydration. This condition causes a shift of fluids from the intracellular compartment to the extracellular, causing cell shrinkage. If severe, dehydration can cause comatose and death.

For example, you are suffering from dehydration and your liver cells are affected. Liver cells are some of the busiest cells in the body. They perform many functions, including detoxification, production of energy and conversion of toxic metabolites to less toxic ones. If liver cells shrink or die due to dehydration, then all these functions will be reduced.

Detoxification is one process that helps in delaying the aging process. It is a process that neutralizes wastes in the body. If the liver cells are unable to perform its job of detoxifying waste products, then more toxins accumulate inside the body and generate more harm to the tissues. The same is true when your body is unable to excrete these harmful metabolites due to dehydration. With less water, the flow of blood becomes slower, which in turn leads to a reduced rate of blood filtration in the kidneys.

2. Eat foods rich in antioxidants, vitamins and minerals.

One of the many signs of aging process is the appearance of various diseases and one way to prevent them is to eat healthy foods. Fruits, vegetables, whole grains and fish meat are just some of the foods that are recommended not only to prevent the onset of age-related diseases, but also to slow the aging process.

Many skin products being advertised nowadays are said to be rich in antioxidants. What people don't know is that there are foods, in fact common foods, that contain great amounts of antioxidants. Vitamin C, Vitamin E and Vitamin A are some of the most potent antioxidants known. They prevent aging by stabilizing the free radicals produced by cellular metabolism.

Vitamin C is found in many citrus fruits like guava, oranges and lemon. Two of the highest sources of this vitamin are pomegranate and kiwi. Be sure to include them in your meals. On the other hand, vitamin E is most commonly found in dark green vegetables, like kale, spinach, broccoli and mustard. Vitamin A, which is known to improve eyesight, is present in yellow and orange fruits and vegetables, like carrots, tomatoes and squash. These three vitamins can promote skin cell renewal and can give you a younger-looking skin.

Another antioxidant found in some fruits and vegetables is resveratrol and lycopene that are both found in tomatoes. These two antioxidants can prevent the occurrence of many forms of cancer and reduce the risk of many cardiovascular diseases, like coronary artery disease and heart attack. Resveratrol is also found in red wine, coffee and grapes. Studies show that a shot of red wine every day can help prevent cardiovascular diseases.

Maintenance of blood pressure is also a major concern in aging. As one ages, the tone of the blood vessels increases causing a rise in the pressure through which the heart must pump blood against. One of the major causes of an increase in blood pressure among old adults is the accumulation of cholesterol in blood vessels. Hence, it is recommended that you eat fiber-rich foods, such as whole grains, wheat, barley and oats. Most fruits and vegetables are also rich in fiber. This indigestible substance prevents aging by lowering the levels of cholesterol in the blood. How does it do that?

Fiber binds bile, a substance that the liver produces to emulsify fats in the diet, and promotes its excretion. Bile, which is mostly made up of cholesterol, is normally recycled and is returned to the gallbladder for storage. Normally, only 2% of the total amount of bile produced by the liver is excreted every day, which means that 98% of it goes back to the circulation. But with fiber, the amount of bile excreted is increased, stimulating the liver to produce more bile. To be able to produce bile, the liver must mobilize and utilize the body's cholesterol stores. This causes the cholesterol blood levels to go down, and eventually, the blood pressure go down, as well.

Blood pressure is also maintained by eating foods rich in omega-3 fatty acids that are most commonly found in fish meat. Fish like salmon, tuna and mackerel are some of the most common and best sources of omega-3. This is a long chain polyunsaturated fatty acid that is easily emulsified in the body. Omega-3 fatty acid is shown to reduce the risk of stroke, hypertension and even Alzheimer's disease.

Aging can also lead to loss of bone mass, which is mainly due to the effect of a decrease in the levels of hormones, such as estrogen. To prevent loss of bone mass, one must eat foods rich in calcium and vitamin D that are found in milk, anchovies, and dairy products, like cheese and butter. However, it is also important to check the labels of the dairy products that you buy. Most of them are also rich in cholesterol. Look for dairy products that do not contain saturated and trans-fats, since these types of fats can solidify inside the blood vessels.

3. Avoid processed, high-fat and sugar-rich foods.

Nowadays, processed foods have become more common, and because of that, the incidence of hypertension, diabetes mellitus and cancer has increased. Most processed foods are rich in chemicals like nitrosamines and benzene that are known to cause various forms of cancer, and sodium, a mineral which is associated with hypertension. Sodium is one of the major electrolytes of the body. However, excessive blood levels of sodium can pull fluids from the intracellular compartment to the intravascular space, or the space inside the vessels, causing an increase in blood volume. This in turn can cause high blood pressure because of the increased workload of the heart.

Sugar-rich foods, on the other hand, can cause diabetes mellitus. Sugars in foods are broken down into glucose inside the body and are then metabolized for the production of energy. Metabolism, as mentioned earlier, generates more free radicals, thus entailing damage to the cells. An increase in glucose in the blood can also lead to diabetes mellitus, a condition characterized by a blood glucose level more than 110 mg/dl, thickening of the blood, and a decrease in blood flow. With slower blood flow, the delivery of oxygen and nutrients to the cells becomes impaired, causing damage.

Fatty foods are rich in cholesterol, which has been said to cause an increase in blood pressure. Accumulation of cholesterol in the blood and deposition of cholesterol into the walls of blood vessels can activate the inflammatory process. Inflammatory cells called neutrophils and macrophages produce chemicals to degrade these cholesterol deposits. Reactions of these chemicals can produce free radicals, and instead of producing beneficial effects to the body by degrading cholesterol, the inflammatory process has, in fact, caused greater harm.

Four Easy Things You Can Do To Prevent Wrinkles

The most visible signs of aging are seen in the skin. The skin gets wrinkled, dry, dark and saggy. Though different skin care products promise a reduction in wrinkles and dark spots, one can never be forever young. You can only delay the aging process, but you cannot stop it. The problem with these skin care products is that not all of them are healthy and not all of them are effective. Some skin care products contain lead, para-aminobenzoic acids and formaldehyde that are all-harmful to the cells and may even be carcinogenic. To avoid the harmful effects of these skin care products, you can try these natural solutions in obtaining a younger-looking skin.

1. Protect your skin from the sun.

The ultraviolet rays emitted by the sun are the culprits of major skin cancers and cellular damage, hence must be avoided. There are three ways on how to protect your skin from the damaging effects of the sun. First, avoid walking or staying under the sun during the peak of UV rays production. UV rays are most intense between 10 am to 4 pm, so it is better to stay at home or limit your exposure to the sun during these hours. Second, use umbrella and wide-brimmed hats when going out. Use UV-protected umbrellas to maximize the protection that you get. Wide-brimmed hats are used for face protection. Your facial skin is very thin, and thus, very sensitive to the damaging effects of the UV rays. Wrinkles and skin darkening are just some of the effects of the UV rays to your face. And third, wear protective clothing. Avoid using dark-colored shirts when staying under the sun. In contrast to light-colored shirts that only reflect the UV rays, dark colors tend to absorb UV rays, and thus, allow them to penetrate to your skin.

2. Get the right amount of sleep.

Cell renewal happens during sleeping hours, and is most effective when the body is relaxed. Lack of sleep can disrupt the renewal process and allows the senescent cells to stay. The skin cells are among the most active cells in the body, renewing every few hours. This means that dead skin cells are continuously shedding off from the body. If cell renewal does not occur and dead skin cells stay, then your skin will become dry. Lack of sleep can also cause formation of dark circles around your eyes. Your skin will lose its natural glow without the right amount of sleep.

If you are having difficulty getting enough sleep, then here are a few tips that you can follow:

- Turn off the lights when sleeping. Aside from helping you get a more comfortable sleep, turning off the lights reduces the risk of cancer. In contrast to what most people know, UV rays are not only produced by the sun. Light bulbs also emit UV rays when turned on. Hence, it is better to turn these lights off when sleeping.
- Avoid eating heavy meals before sleeping. Large meals can cause abdominal pain and acid reflux when you lie down. These discomforts can prevent you from getting a good night sleep.
- Avoid drinking plenty of water at night. Drinking too much water before going to bed can disrupt your sleep pattern as the frequency of urination increases. Drink a lot of water during the day instead.
- Relax and avoid worrying once you lie down on your bed. Worries can keep you awake all night, thus must be put aside when you retire to bed.

3. Use natural scrubs, moisturizers and exfoliates for your skin.

Extracts of some fruits and vegetables can be used as scrubs on your skin. Choose those that are rich in antioxidants, like lemon, orange, oats and tea. You can mix sugar and lemon juice or tea to create a facial scrub. Sugar crystals help peel away dead skin cells while the juice or the tea provides antioxidants for your skin. Exfoliation does not only remove the dead skin cells on the surface of your skin, but also allows the antioxidants and moisturizers to penetrate the skin better.

You can also moisturize your skin without the use of the common skin care products out there. Almond oil and avocadoes can be used as moisturizers due to their fat content. You may be alarmed that these foods are rich in fats but you have nothing to worry. Almonds and avocadoes contain good fats including omega-3 fatty acids and HDL. Mix 3 tablespoons of almond oil and a half-cup of avocado until smooth. Apply this on your face for 30 minutes and rinse. You can do this every night for better results.

4. Protect your hands from drying.

Your hands serve as your calling card. Even if you have received Botox treatments for your face and neck, you cannot deny the wrinkles on your hands. Your hands can give information about your age, so it is better to protect them from the aging process, as well. Aside from avoiding exposure to harsh chemicals, you can use some fruit extracts to create a simple homemade moisturizer for your hands. You can mix orange or lemon, honey and uncooked rice to create a hand scrub. The uncooked rice serves as exfoliate, lemon or orange helps lighten your skin and keep it radiant, while honey smoothens your skin.

FITNESS TIPS TO PREVENT AGING

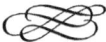

"Fitness is a youth serum."

-Maureen Hagan

Exercise does a lot of beneficial things to the body- it prevents cardiovascular diseases, keeps your muscles in shape, keeps your bones strong, stimulates the release of endogenous opioids to make you feel better and facilitates the movement of various vitamins and minerals inside the body. What most people don't know is that exercise is also a way of slowing down the aging process. It does not only make you look younger, but it makes you feel younger, as well.

WHAT HAPPENS IN EXERCISE? While most people perform exercises as a way of toning their muscles up and achieving a body-to-die-for, exercise actually gives you something more. As your muscles move during exercise, your blood is more efficiently pumped back to the heart. While it is true that the heart pumps the blood into circulation, it is also a fact that it needs help in getting the huge volume of blood to return to the heart. It gets the help it needs from the muscles of the body. The muscles, especially those in the lower extremities, serve as secondary mechanical pumps that push the blood back to the heart by 'squeezing' the blood vessels periodically. This improves blood flow into the different areas of the body, which in turn enhances the delivery of oxygen and nutrients to the cells. The organs receive the nutrients they need and they get to efficiently perform their functions.

EXERCISE ALSO PROMOTES the release of Beta-endorphins, which are endogenous chemicals that bind to opioid receptors in the body. These chemicals enhance your feeling of well-being and relieve stress. This is the reason why you feel good and energetic after doing some exercises.

EXERCISE CAN ALSO PREVENT diabetes mellitus by promoting glucose uptake in cells. Diabetes mellitus is known to be caused by an increase in the blood glucose levels, which may either be due to a resistance to insulin or a decrease in its production. Insulin is a hormone that promotes metabolism of glucose and its production is enhanced by exercise. As you exercise, more and more glucose molecules leave the bloodstream and are used up by cells for energy production.

WHAT IS SO surprising about exercise is that it can actually slow the progression of aging. It has already been mentioned that exercise promotes blood flow, which corresponds to an increase in the rate of waste excretion. With more toxins being excreted, the cells can regenerate faster. An increase in blood flow can also promote the growth of collagen and proliferation of elastin that are all needed for healthy skin. Collagen serves as the foundation of any cell, while elastin keeps your skin resistant to trauma. These two substances also prevent the development of wrinkles.

Following these simple fitness guide can reduce the risks of diseases and can delay the signs of aging.

1. Do brisk walking every day.

Many experts say that walking is the best exercise. Taking 10,000 steps a day is proven to reduce the risk of cardiovascular diseases, such as atherosclerosis, heart failure and heart attack. Brisk walking is a type of an aerobic exercise. This type of exercise makes use of oxygen as the substrate for the production of energy and is considered to be more beneficial than the anaerobic type. Anaerobic exercises result to production of lactic acid, which is mainly responsible for muscle cramping and metabolic disturbances.

2. Perform squatting exercises.

One of the most common musculoskeletal signs of aging is

the inflammation of weight-bearing joints, such as the knees and hips. These joints become inflamed because of the loss of the synovial fluid that cushions the bones forming the joints. As the amount of synovial fluid decreases, the bones forming the joints become more prone to friction, which eventually leads to inflammation. This process produces joint pains, wherein older individuals experience difficulty picking up something from the floor, difficulty climbing stairs and difficulty raising their legs. To prevent these from happening and to stabilize the joints more firmly, squatting exercises can be performed. Try squatting from your knees for 10 times every day, resting for 5 seconds in between each squat and holding each squatting position for 10 seconds. Squatting helps align your bones, strengthen your joints and prevent joint pains.

3. Practice Yoga regularly.

Yoga has been known to be an exercise that facilitates weight loss and an exercise that keeps your body in good shape. However, there is more to yoga than that. Yoga, in most part, works like meditation. It is used for mind relaxation, relieving you of your stressors and worries by the power of concentration. It also enhances one's flexibility by assuming various positions in order to facilitate breathing. Yoga is now also used as an exercise to delay aging.

Older individuals have slower metabolic rate than the younger population, which means that their ability to produce energy and convert toxic products into less toxic metabolites are impaired or reduced. This is where yoga comes in. Yoga incorporates deep breathing exercises that facilitate the flow of oxygen through the different parts of the body. With more oxygen being delivered, the cells have more substrates for energy production and metabolism is increased. Yoga also helps improve balance and may be beneficial to older people who are at risk of falling or slipping, thus may prevent injuries.

THE SECRET TO KEEPING YOUR MIND YOUNG & HEALTHY

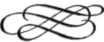

"You don't stop laughing when you grow old, you grow old when you stop laughing."

-George Bernard Shaw

Many people say that youth is a state of mind, and so is aging. Someday, when you have grown older, the visible signs of aging will fill your face and skin and you can't do anything about it. But there is such a thing as graceful aging. This does not refer to the beauty of your skin or to the strength of your muscles or bones when you age; rather, it refers to your attitude towards aging. Do you feel positive about getting old or do you feel like it's the end of the world for you?

Not everyone can embrace aging as other people can. There are people who are very skeptic about it and consider aging as a process of deterioration. But there are also some people who think of it as a process of maturation and gaining more wisdom. The more you try to avoid aging and the more you worry about it, the more you age. Aging, as mentioned in the first few chapters of the book, is something that is expected and universal. No one is exempted from it. What you can only do is to delay the process, but not totally stop it.

Your attitude plays a major role in the aging process. Staying positive and enthusiastic about your future despite the wrinkling of your skin, the greying and thinning out of your hair, and the weakening of your bones creates a great difference in your life. You may have all these visible signs of aging, but they don't matter when you have youthful thinking.

Thinking positively can delay aging in many ways. First, it decreases your anxiety. When you think that there is something good behind all the negative things that you are going through, you will stop worrying about unnecessary things. Instead of wallowing in misery because you know that you are not getting any younger, why not enjoy the moments that you have with your family and friends? In contrast to the belief of many that aging gives you less time to enjoy your life, aging actually does the opposite! Now that you are retired from work and you have all the time in the world, this is the best time to enjoy and have fun!

Second, thinking positively can improve your resistance against diseases. How does this happen? Thinking positively lessens the stress that you feel, which in turn, lessens the release of certain hormones that respond to stressful situations. One of your stress hormones is cortisol, a glucocorticoid produced by the adrenal glands. Cortisol, just like any other steroids, is an immunosuppressant that prevents stimulation of cells involved in one's immunity. This means that the more you are stressed, the more you produce cortisol; and the more you produce cortisol, the less able you are to fight off infections and diseases. Cortisol can also augment the release of other hormones, such as epinephrine and norepinephrine that are involved in sympathetic stimulation. Sympathetic stimulation results to an increase in blood pressure and resistance to the effects of insulin, predisposing one to hypertension and diabetes mellitus.

And lastly, thinking positively gives you more freedom. It frees you from the limitations of aging that most people are worried about. When you think positively, you don't think about your bones being decalcified, or your skin being saggy and wrinkled. Being optimistic can make you do more- it can make you socialize more with friends and it can make you accomplish more things.

Here are some ways on how you can keep a positive and youthful attitude:

1. Laugh more often.

Laughing makes use of fewer muscles than frowning, which means that there is less energy needed to smile than to frown. Try to make it your habit to post a smile on your face. Smiling lifts the muscles of your face up and prevents it from sagging. Aside from that laughter can take away your worries. Laughter can promote the release of serotonin, a neurotransmitter that is involved in regulation of your mood. This neurotransmitter is also called a happy hormone because it can enhance the feeling of well-being.

2. Be grateful with what you are.

Being appreciative of what you are and being thankful for it is a sign of acceptance of the aging process. When you become grateful, you get to focus on your blessings and all the beautiful things that are happening to you right now. Be grateful for the sun for it gives you hope. Be grateful for your age for it means that you have lived long. Be grateful for waking up this morning for it gives you another chance to enjoy your life.

3. Socialize with your friends and family.

Spending time and bonding with your loved ones is one

of the best ways on how to keep a positive attitude towards aging. When you are with them, you tend to forget about your age and your diseases. All you can feel is that you are loved, you are appreciated and that you are accepted no matter who you are and no matter how old you are.

4. Keep doing what you love.

Most people hate aging because they feel like they can't do the things that they used to do anymore. They cannot drive, stitch and dance the way they used to when they were young. Growing old should not limit you from doing what you want; rather, it should motivate you to live your passion. Dance with your friends, join a knitting club and go see a movie with your family.

AFTERWORD

Aging is not all about the physical changes that happen when you grow old; rather it is also about how you perceive and accept it. Perceiving aging as a positive event in your life helps you cope with it easily. Old age-related diseases are given, as well as the decline in your physical and mental abilities. What you can control is your reaction to aging. If you think that there's nothing good about aging, then you will spend the rest of your days in despair. You will only stress yourself out and deprive yourself of happiness. If you think that you have become wiser and better with age, then congratulate yourself - you have just slowed down aging! Eating healthy foods, performing exercises, taking care of your skin and thinking positively can absolutely make you look younger and live longer!

www.ingramcontent.com/pod-product-compliance
Lightning Source LLC
Chambersburg PA
CBHW070038040426
42333CB00040B/1716